Compassionate Town Planning

GORDON STEPHENSON

Edited by Hugh Stretton

with a Preface by Gordon Cherry

ESS

Preface

Gordon Stephenson, born in 1908, is one of the few remaining 20th century figures, happily still with us today, who can speak with authority about, and with personal recollections of, the great planning events of our time. Friend of William Holford and co-worker with Patrick Abercrombie, he helped to shape the British post-war planning system. For six years, from 1948, he was Lever Professor of Civic Design in the University of Liverpool and Editor of the *Town Planning Review*. Rebuffed from taking up a chair at MIT, he established a city planning school at Toronto. He subsequently transferred his affections to Australia, where he took the Foundation Chair of Architecture at the University of Western Australia in 1960. His autobiography, *On a Human Scale*, was published in 1992.

His present monograph is a compelling read – for its insights as well as its biases. Its very title gives the game away: what young professional today would talk about 'compassionate planning'? But for Gordon Stephenson town planning was precisely that – a humanitarian corrective to the urban degradation of yester-year, driven by a belief that squalor could be eradicated from industrial towns and cities and that dignity and beauty could be restored to them for the lasting benefit of human kind. It was a compelling vision, and if we today have lost it, then we are the poorer for it.

The monograph is a personal statement. He shares his generation's belief that the emergent town planning movement around the turn of the last century, fed by radical reformism, could sustain the uplifting march from Coketown to Utopia. He demonstrates an eclectic interest in all forms of town building, wherever it is to be found; Adelaide emerges as a civilised guide-post. He tells us of his work for the Greater London Plan and in developing 'planning techniques' for the post-war system. He offers rare vignettes of people with whom he came into contact. He comments (unfavourably) on the very different world of today in which town planning now finds itself.

For these reasons the monograph is a period piece. It tells us almost as much about Gordon Stephenson as he tells us about 20th century town planning. The profession, in Britain at least, can boast few today who share his qualities; we seem to have squeezed out the polymath, the well-read, the historically informed, those curious about city form and structure as they change over time, and those driven by a view about future society and human relations. The author was (and is) all these things, with an ability to make relationships between knowledge and experiences in a lifelong crusade of conviction and purpose.

It is a contemporary regret, not a weakness of his past judgement, that his vision of planning, which was humane and compassionate, seems unrealisable in today's world. It is a challenge for another generation to work out a new framework for town planning in harmony with societal aspirations, economic systems and political institutions. In the meantime we have much to learn from the career of an international practitioner; we can read his many reflections with both instruction and delight.

Gordon E. Cherry
Emeritus Professor of Urban and Regional Planning
University of Birmingham

Contents

The Nineteenth Century

There is much to be learned from many centuries of history but it can be said that twentieth century town planning has its roots in the nineteenth century, when the industrial revolution brought about a massive flow of people from the countryside into rapidly growing cities and towns. The degradation of the human condition was appalling, with people crowded into insanitary dwellings and dying in their thousands during a series of epidemics.

In 1844, Friedrich Engels, at the age of 24, and already successfully launched on a business career in Manchester, published his book on the condition of the working classes in England. A year later, Benjamin Disraeli, in his novel Sybil, saw England as "two nations, between whom there is no intercourse and no sympathy; who are as ignorant of each other's habits, thoughts and feelings as if they were dwellers in different zones, or inhabitants of different planets; who are formed by a different breeding, and fed by a different food, and ordered by different manners, and are not governed by the same laws."

Disraeli later became the Tory Prime Minister who had Queen Victoria crowned as Empress of India. His comparison of the rich and the poor was written as if to amplify the pertinent observations of Engels when he described a Manchester slum in which "all drains and refuse find their way in to the (river) Irk, which receives further the contents of all the neighbouring sewers and privies...Below the bridge you look upon the piles of debris, the refuse, filth and offal from the courts on the steep left bank. Here each house is packed close behind its neighbour and a piece of each is visible, all black, smoky, crumbling, ancient, with broken panes, and window frames...The background is furnished by old barrack-like factory buildings...and embraces the pauper burial ground, the workhouse, the 'Poor Law Bastille of Manchester', which like a citadel looks threateningly down upon the working people's quarters below."

Professor Patrick Abercrombie once said "The whole of the nineteenth century outburst of town-building was likened by

Cobbett, who was living in the midst of it, to an epidemic of wens, with London as the GREAT WEN. And the wen, though it depends on human sustenance, is beyond human control." Born in 1763, William Cobbett, the political writer, fought the evils and squalor of capitalist cities all his life. But unbridled economic laissez-faire was the order of the day. As Catherine Bauer put it "With Malthus and Ricardo for text, a whole system of common ideology was evolved to rationalise the existence of a large class condemned to living in a slum." Marx and Engels said that big cities were bad and would gradually disappear under socialism. By the end of the century Ebenezer Howard was proposing how they could be restrained and reshaped under capitalism.

During the nineteenth century, a growing number of the more fortunate members of society, motivated by compassion, conscience or fear, pressed for reform through parliamentary or local government action. The first association for housing reform, the Society for Bettering the Condition of the Poor, had been formed in 1797, with William Wilberforce one of the protagonists. In Parliament, ten years later, he successfully promoted his Abolition of Slavery Bill. It was not until 1844 that the first Royal Commission on Health and Housing was appointed, the year of Friedrich Engel's book on the condition of the working classes.

The Hungry and Insanitary Forties

In 1848, the first Public Health Act was passed. It was the year of the Chartist Riots, Continental revolutions, and the first editions of John Stuart Mill's *Principles of Political Economy* and the *Communist Manifesto* by Karl Marx and Friedrich Engels.

According to Catherine Bauer (Bauer, 1934), the 1848 Public Health Act was "the first piece of positive housing legislation in modern history." 1848 also witnessed the outbreak of a cholera epidemic which in 1850 carried off more than 50,000 men, women and children. Four years earlier, as if preparing itself for the worst outbreak of cholera, the City of Liverpool had appointed Dr Duncan as the first Medical Officer of Health in Britain, and probably the world.

Before his appointment, Dr William Duncan had for ten years been attached to the Liverpool Dispensaries. In 1843, in a lecture to the Liverpool Literary and Philosophical Society, he described the loathsome condition of people crowded into rows of tiny back to back houses facing narrow courts, with a common standpipe and privy at the end of each court. He knew of one court with a population of one person per square yard, and an area of courtyard housing at a density of 600,000 persons per square mile. He said "even these figures of overcrowding, terrible as they are, do not quite plumb the depths of misery and degradation in which the casual labourers and their families had to live at that period" (Simey, 1992).

During the industrial revolution, immigrants were pouring into the towns from the countryside and Ireland. In his first annual report, Dr Duncan wrote "The 1st of January, 1847, found this pauper immigration steadily increasing, and it continued in such rapidly progressive rates, that by the end of June not less than 300,000 Irish had landed in Liverpool. Of these it was very moderately estimated that from 60,000 to 80,000 had located themselves among us, occupying every nook and cranny of the already overcrowded lodging-houses, and forcing their way into cellars (about 3,000 in number) which had been closed under the provisions of the Health Act, 1842. In different parts of Liverpool 50 or 60 of these destitute people were found in a house containing three or four small rooms, about 12 feet by 10; and in more than one instance upwards of 40 were found sleeping in a cellar" (Frazer, 1947).

Nationally, in terms of public health, (Sir) Edwin Chadwick (1800-1890) was the dominant influence. In 1834, he was appointed Secretary to the Poor Laws Commission. In 1842, he completed a close examination of the Boards of Guardians' medical records and produced a damning indictment of the sanitary conditions of the labouring population. Two years later, with Dr Southward Smith and others, he completed *The Health of Towns Report for the House of Commons.* This demonstrated the urgent need for adequate sanitation, unpolluted water supply, and the appointment of supervisory authorities employing engineering and medical specialists. It led to the Public Health Act of 1848, the year in which Dr John Simon was appointed the first Medical Officer of Health in London.

Sir Edwin Chadwick and a growing number of other reformers lived long enough to see Parliament pass the great Public Health Act of 1875, enacted during Disraeli's second term as Prime Minister. The provisions covered pollution, the regulation of streets, highways and new buildings, daylighting and ventilation of dwellings, the removal of nuisances, the inspection of food, the regulation of markets and sanitary burial. Both the 1848 and 1875 Acts received impetus from the writings of the Poet Laureate, Robert Southey (1774-1845) and a growing number of novelists, including Mrs Elizabeth Gaskell (1810-1865) and Charles Dickens (1812-1870). Between 1875 and the First World War, grid-iron layouts of bye-law housing prevailed in nearly all new suburbs and provided what Osbert Lancaster described as "salubrious dwellings for industrious artisans" (Lancaster, 1939).

A concern to protect the people's health thus generated some practical steps toward planning their cities.

Origins of Modern Planning

The 1848 Public Health Act signalled the beginning of the end of the insanitary forties. It coincided with the early days of the great cholera epidemic, which was raging in 1849 when James Silk Buckingham published his *National Evils and Practical Remedies,* portraying in great detail an ideal new town, Victoria. In 1850, a year later, and at the height of the cholera epidemic, Ebenezer Howard was born in the City of London. His parents and others would no doubt tell him about the epidemic and Cobbett's Great Wen spreading malignantly into the East End docklands.

Before the end of the century Howard had written *Tomorrow: a Peaceful Path to Real Reform* in which he reached conclusions from the work and ideas of nineteenth century reformers, and showed how Buckingham's idea of building a new town could be achieved. Shortly after the publication of the third edition, retitled *Garden Cities of Tomorrow* (Howard, 1902), Letchworth, the First Garden City, was started by a Joint Stock Company he had formed. It heralded a succession of twentieth century new towns planned and developed by either public or private corporations in different parts of the world. Howard was an important link between nineteenth and twentieth century planning. But he also was able to build on the work of predecessors. Two earlier contributions had been specially influential: the work of Robert Owen, and the colonial town-planning that had been inspired by the ideas of the first generation of Utilitarians or Philosophical Radicals.

The Ideals and Ideas of Robert Owen

A younger contemporary of Cobbett and Wilberforce, Robert Owen (1771-1858), made the first statement of problems in the industrial world. In *Modern Housing* Catherine Bauer described Owen as a "man who combined in one remarkable person all the characteristics of a moral reformer, a doctrinaire socialist, a romantic utopian experimenter, a practical sociologist, an earnest statesman, a labour organiser, an enlightened employer and a successful self-made business man" (Bauer, 1934).

Owen carried out many reforms in New Lanark, Scotland, where he had in 1800 established a successful cotton mill. He was well known in the business world as having increased dividends through shortening working hours, paying higher wages, and providing education, better working and living conditions and wages during slack periods. Because of his views, he was invited some years later to address the American Congress.

After the Battle of Waterloo, Britain suffered a severe economic depression. Owen's words concerning the crisis of 1816 were: "The want of hands and raw materials (during the war), with this lavish expenditure, created a demand for the great encouragement to new mechanical inventions and chemical discoveries, to supersede manual labour. The war was a great and extravagant customer...And on the day when peace was signed, this great customer of the producers died, and prices fell as the demands diminished...The barns and farmyards were full, warehouses loaded, and such was our artificial state of society, that this very superabundance of wealth was the sole cause of the existing distress."

The post-war depression of 1816 caused Owen to propose a plan that would provide cooperative communities for the unemployed, who would work in both industry and agriculture and become self-supporting. Public funds for poor relief and workhouses would not be required and children would benefit from education and a decent environment. Owen was a man of influence and at first his plan received considerable support.

Newspapers, including *The Times*, printed his report in full, and economists, including Ricardo, saw it as a new form of charitable relief (Bauer, 1934).

He presented his plan to the Parliamentary Committee on the Poor Law in 1817, together with a drawing, a description of the buildings and the layout, and a complete financial statement. There is no evidence that the Committee gave his plan serious consideration, but he is credited with having instigated the Factory Act of 1819.

Owen died in 1858, at the age of 87, having lived long enough to see many social and economic changes and the beginning of modern town planning. He remained active, and eventually anticipated the socialists of the early twentieth century in advocating public ownership of land and means of production, equalised consumption, and continuous socio-economic analysis in decision making. He witnessed the first conscious uprising of an urban proletariat in the Chartist movement and would have known most of the parliamentary followers of the philosopher, Jeremy Bentham.

The Utilitarians or Philosophical Radicals

A milestone in the development of parliamentary democracy was reached in 1832, the year in which the Reform Bill, prepared by Earl Grey's Whig Government, redistributed House of Commons seats in the interest of larger communities and gave the franchise to middle class men. In the reformed Parliament of 1833, the followers of the philosopher Jeremy Bentham "wielded, by reason of the forcefulness of their ideas an influence on the legislation of the thirties out of all proportion to their numbers" (Hyde, 1947).

In 1838 the national Chartist movement submitted to Viscount Melbourne's Government a charter containing six demands for further reform: 1) abolition of property qualifications for MPs; 2) manhood suffrage; 3) ballot voting; 4) equal electoral districts; 5) payment of MPs; 6) annual parliaments.

In 1789, six years after the Treaty of Paris ended the American Revolution, and during the French Revolution, Jeremy Bentham had enunciated the theory of "utility" in his *Introduction to Principles of Morals and Legislation.* In it he evolved the "greatest happiness" principle that government should be activated to benefit the greatest number in all forms of social activity. Bentham died in 1832. By then the leading exponents of his doctrine of utility were John Stuart Mill and John Arthur Roebuck. Mill became the progenitor of subsequent liberal thought in supplementing utilitarianism with humanitarian principles, in which pleasure as a motivating force should be measured by quality as well as quantity.

According to the economic historian, Francis Hyde, John Arthur Roebuck was the Utilitarian who contributed most to town planning theory. "He had himself experienced a carefree upbringing, and from the age of thirteen had lived in Canada, where the broad rivers, the vast primeval forests and the mountains had had a profound effect on his mental development...The state of the towns and the conditions under which the working classes lived appalled him...His natural aversion to town life and habits was heightened when he saw the vice, the disease and the social disorganisation within the towns. To reform such conditions was, to him, not merely a matter of expedients, it was fundamentally a question of education and town reconstruction; education to quicken the public conscience to the enormity of the evils, and reconstruction through direct parliamentary action..." (Hyde, 1947).

As early as 1828, when the enclosure of common land around the towns was going on, Roebuck "had outlined a programme of town planning and town development in accordance with Benthamite principles...He had advocated tree-lined boulevards, grass lawns open to the public, and flower-bedecked parks; while outside the towns, and if possible ringing them round, large tracts of common land varying in size according to population and maintained by the town authorities or by the State itself for town dwellers." He said "We must create a public trust and prevent by law if necessary the rights of the common people from being swept away at the hand of the proprietor who would enclose the land round our towns for his own future profit, and the pseudo-builder who would cover it with ugliness." Speaking of the worker in a pamphlet published in 1835, Roebuck wrote "You will not let him dance or hear music; you do all you can to put an end to his cricket and bowls; you shut him out of the green fields; you drive him from the common; you close the Picture Gallery and the Museum on feast days and holidays, but you leave open the gin and the beer-shop; hating convivial meetings you make the people unsocial drunkards."

In 1836, when Viscount Melbourne was Prime Minister in the reformed parliament, the Philosophical Radicals managed to attach an important clause to a Common Field Enclosure Bill which exempted common fields from enclosure if they came within a certain radius of the big towns. The radii varied, according to the size of the town, from a radius of one mile for a town of 5,000 inhabitants to a radius of ten miles for London. Although Viscount Melbourne remained Prime Minister after the election of 1837, the philosophical radicals suffered catastrophic defeat and Roebuck lost his seat. In the election of 1841, the Tories under Sir Robert Peel were returned to power, and although Roebuck was re-elected he was almost alone in trying to save land for the needs of town populations. But his ideas lived on and were put into effect in the planning of colonial towns and the establishment of mid-nineteenth century town parks.

The two most important planning achievements resulting from the parliamentary activity of the Utilitarians were the provision of nineteenth century public parks in Britain, its colonies, and indirectly the USA, and the planning and settlement of new towns and their surrounding agricultural hinterlands in Australia and New Zealand. The latter were largely due to the organising ability of Edward Gibbon Wakefield, influenced by Jeremy Bentham, who had strongly opposed colonisation through convict transportation.

Colonial Planning

Edward Gibbon Wakefield (1796-1862) was an outstanding figure in the planning of colonial settlements and towns. His family had a long association with Jeremy Bentham, whose followers, the Utilitarians, were aware that colonisation had stagnated after the loss of the thirteen American colonies, but was once more proceeding apace. Their interest in colonisation was that it provided testing grounds for their social and legislative projccts. Many Utilitarians became members of the National Colonisation Society, which advanced the systematic colonisation of Australia and New Zealand.

In modern terms, Wakefield would be classed as an entrepreneur as well as a persuasive writer and organiser. At the age of 30 he took part in an abduction and was imprisoned in Newgate for three years (1826-29). During his enforced leisure time he began researching colonisation. Imprisonment "by shutting him out from a wide range of activity channelled his energies and multiplied the force of his personality." In prison he not only had time to read and think but also had contact with men and women who were the raw material of British colonisation.

Shortly before he left prison, Wakefield wrote his famous *Letter from Sydney* in which he played the role of a fictitious settler, who was critical of the general disorder and lack of direction in the colony of New South Wales. At that time, "some seven million acres of land had been alienated, yet the free settlers numbered only some forty thousand, most of them living at the level of subsistence." Wakefield showed that giving away colonial land or selling it for next to nothing was a hindrance and not a help to colonisation.

In 1831, Wakefield persuaded Bentham to edit his project for colonisation and to write one of his last pamphlets, *Emancipate your Colonies.* In 1833, Wakefield published his *England and America,* which included an appendix of "The Art of Colonisation." The final version of *The Art of Colonisation,* was published in 1849. It set out the principles he had enunciated for establishing settlements and new towns in the colonies (Wakefield, 1849).

At the end of the century Ebenezer Howard quoted Wakefield at great length (*Garden Cities of Tomorrow,* 1902) putting forward similar arguments for new towns in the United Kingdom. Howard also reminded his readers that the Ancient Greeks in establishing new colonies through necessity "*sent out a representation of the parent State – colonists from all ranks.*" This was the essence of Wakefield's thesis.

Wakefield argued that colonies used as dumping grounds for convicts and paupers repelled industrious men and women seeking better opportunities for themselves and their children; and that the hardships and risks of emigration could be mitigated by well planned organisation. The latter would include land surveyed before it was sold, and the selection of emigrants so that there was a reasonable balance of sexes, age groups and occupations. The Wakefield system incorporated the doctrine of a "fixed, uniform and sufficient price" for land tenure in the colonies.

"In an England growing conscious of the squalor and misery of the industrial towns, it was natural that men should turn to the empty territories of the new world as an outlet for a seemingly redundant population." (Hight and Straubel, 1957).

With the backing of the Philosophical Radicals, Wakefield proved to be a conspicuous leader in the mid-nineteenth century colonisation of Australia, New Zealand and Canada. As early as 1831 he persuaded John Stuart Mill, Jeremy Bentham, Col. Robert Torrens and others to join him in founding the South Australian Land Company. Torrens as a member of the Company's Committee of Enquiry had discussions with Robert Owen before the Company failed. Not to be outdone, and realising that the Government must be brought in, the South Australian Association was formed in 1833 to seek a charter and the assistance of the Duke of Wellington. In 1834, when Sir Robert Peel was Tory Prime Minister, the Iron Duke introduced legislation in the House of Lords which granted land to the Association. The Act was passed in August, 1834, "to empower His Majesty (William IV) to erect South Australia into a British Province or Provinces and to provide for the colonisation and government thereof."

Adelaide: A Milestone in Planning History

With the mother country in the throes and horrors of the industrial revolution, British town planning was at its best in the colonies. Encapsulating the ideas of the Philosophical Radicals, Wakefield and other reformers, Adelaide was sited and planned by Colonel William Light in 1836. It has proved to be a milestone in planning history.

In any age, Light would have been perceived as a gifted person. Early in life he would be influenced by his father. In 1786, the year after he was born to a part Malay mother, his father, Captain Francis Light, working for the British East India Company, founded Prince of Wales Island (now Penang) in the British Strait Settlement. He also planned the capital, Georgetown, of which the historic centre is now an important and unique architectural heritage. Established to control the spice route through the Strait of Malacca, the settlement quickly became a multicultural society which included Arabs, Armenians, Chinese, strait-born Chinese, Eurasians, Europeans, Javanese, Jews, Indians, Malays, Persians and Sumatrans.

In England William Light was in turn a midshipman in the Royal Navy and an officer in the Dragoons. As a dashing cavalry officer in the Peninsular War (1808-1812) he was promoted Colonel by Sir Arthur Wellesley (later the Duke of Wellington). He would be remembered by the Iron Duke when, at his instigation, the South Australian Association was granted land in 1834.

After the Napoleonic Wars, Light married Mary, a natural daughter of the Duke of Richmond. For a long period they wandered the Mediterranean in their yacht, when he further developed his skills as a navigator, and in sketching landscapes and cities. Mary left him for his friend. Years later he was to die in the arms of Maria Gandy, a Suffolk woman, with whom he had shared his life in Adelaide. After three and a half years of triumph and disaster he died of tuberculosis, the after effects of a severe wound from the battle of Corunna, and a weakened heart caused by overwork. He had been deeply moved by the pristine beauty of the Australian landscape and had produced an outstanding plan, but he died grievously harmed through the intrigues of narrow minded officials and settlers.

Following Wakefield's precept, the 1834 (South Australia) Act was to establish a double government. The Crown appointed officers and framed laws, and the Colonisation Commission raised money, managed land sales and promoted emigration. The Commission was gazetted in May, 1835, and quickly offered for sale 437 lots at £81 each, entitling the purchaser to one town acre lot in Adelaide and one country section of eighty acres. When more than half the lots were unsold the price was dropped to 12/– per acre and the country sections were increased to 138 acres.

With land selling slowly "one of the commissioners, Angas, formed a joint stock company to take up the remaining land orders...To the confusion of double government was added a powerful representative of capitalism." (Hutchings and Bunker, 1986). Raymond Bunker's chapter two, in their book The Early Years, is an excellent concise history of the founding of Adelaide. The Angas name is perpetuated by Angas Downs, a large land holding in the Northern Territory and Angaston, a delightful town in South Australia's Barossa Valley. By the second half of the nineteenth century a notable gentry had been formed, who styled the colony the "Province of South Australia" to set it apart from the convict ones to the east and west. During the last three decades of the nineteenth century, they promoted contemporary arts and design, supported William Morris's design company and built a seemly city. It is not surprising that Adelaide University was the third to be established in Australia, the Art Gallery is richly endowed, and occasionally it exhibits the drawings and paintings of Colonel William Light.

Light might well have been appointed the first Governor of South Australia. Late in 1834, he was recommended for the post by Sir Charles Napier. He mentioned this to Captain John Hindmarsh, a naval officer, who lobbied the powers that be and was appointed instead. Hindmarsh immediately asked for Light to be made Surveyor-General. They worked together uneasily for less than two years, with Light not only more far-seeing but also the stronger character. Fortunately, in a letter of instruction issued in London on 9 March, 1836, the Colonisation Commissioners gave Light sole responsibility for selecting the site.

Light landed in Australia on 20 August, 1836, and Hindmarsh arrived four months later. Following the explicit instructions of the Commissioners, Light had already explored the considerable coast shown in the map accompanying the instructions (Hutchings and Bunker, 1986), and had made up his mind that the capital city should be in the vicinity of its present location. Being a naval man, Hindmarsh had assumed it should be a port, but Light reminded him that site selection as well as town planning, was his perogative.

Light described the position and form of the city in a sketch surrounded by numerous notes. This was approved at a meeting of settlers on 10 February 1837. Light with his several surveyors had begun to survey the town acres on 11 January, and completed the work on 10 March. Argument about the site continued throughout the year. Light resigned in December, 1837, ill and worn out through overwork and faction fighting. He went into private practice, but just before he died on 6 October, 1839, he wrote.

> The reasons that led me to fix Adelaide where it is I do not expect to be generally understood or calmly judged of at present. My enemies, however, have done me the good service of fixing the whole of the responsibility upon me. I am perfectly willing to bear it, and leave it to posterity and not to them to decide whether I am entitled to praise or blame. (Preface, *A Brief Journal.*)

The vacillating Hindmarsh was succeeded by Governor Gawler. If Light had not been ill, he might have reinstated him after his successor, George Kingston, had shown himself to be far less competent. Light had called Kingston "a vulgar, overbearing upstart." Unfortunately, Light's papers were burned in a fire. Kingston not only outlived him but took far more credit than he deserved and was eventually knighted.

Light had absorbed the philosophy of the Benthamites and acted in response to Wakefield's organising ability. He epitomised the work of new town planners of every epoch, and not only influenced Ebenezer Howard but also the architect-planners of Stevenage, the 1946 prototype of the British New Towns. Even more remarkable, his plan for Adelaide, now the centre of a metropolitan region is as workable, flexible and handsome as it ever was, and is both an encouragement and challenge to present day planners in South Australia.

Every time there is an international cricket match on the oval in Adelaide's Parklands it is televised to Commonwealth Countries in which cricket is played. Invariably, from time to time, the commentators extol the beauty of the cricket ground and its setting, show Colonel Light's statue overlooking the Parklands and the City Centre, and describe Adelaide as their favourite city. When one recalls that Light prepared his plan in a few months, it is a reminder that he was an altogether remarkable man.

Because of the loss of his papers we shall never know the origin of the thoughts and ideas which were in Light's mind when he was siting and planning Adelaide. As a master mariner he would be familiar with surveying instruments, and no doubt during his army career with the work of the Royal Engineers. He was also an artist, interested in landscapes, towns and cities, a sensitive geomorphologist and would be familiar with Roebuck's advocacy of parklands surrounding towns, first promulgated in the British Parliament in 1828. He would also be conscious of the way in which the Renaissance had transformed city building.

Origins of Colonial Town Plans

During the Renaissance, the *Ten Books on Architecture,* written by Vitruvius in the first century B.C., were first translated in 1476. This stimulated creative thinking, and provided a basis for books extending the theory of architecture as the art of city design. In his *Design of Cities,* Edmund Bacon suggests that *l'Architettura,* a book by Cataneo, first published in Venice in 1567, was the origin of a rectilinear town plan with a large central square, and four quarters each containing a lesser square (Bacon, 1967). Light might not have been aware of Cataneo's concept, but very likely he would have seen derivatives in Newcourt's plan for London after the Great Fire of 1666, and Oglethorpe's plan for Savannah, Georgia, 1733.

Cataneo's plan, and those for Philadelphia and Adelaide, adopted the strict orientation of Roman colonial towns built around the major cross-town streets, the *Cardo* and *Decumanus,* and formalised the concept of *quartiers,* or quarters, which had grown organically in medieval and renaissance cities such as Paris and Venice.

In September, 1666, four-fifths of the City of London was destroyed by fire. Of the several quickly presented reconstruction plans a youthful Christopher Wren's baroque extravaganza is the best known. The more practical concept of Richard Newcourt, the Elder, was for long overlooked. He, perhaps better than any other person, understood the anatomy of the City. After having surveyed it and the immediate surrounds, he had published a map of London in 1658, eight years before the Great Fire. According to the historian, T.F. Reddaway, "his map of London was far the best then in existence" (Reddaway, 1939). Newcourts map of 1658 showed that the medieval City consisted of a fairly rectilinear layout of roads, lanes and alleys, with the parish churches and a gothic St Paul's Cathedral acting as focal points.

Amongst the various planning proposals for the reconstruction of the City, Newcourt's responded more to the medieval layout. He prepared two plans, both rectilinear, the second having fewer and larger parishes. Newcourt superimposed his second plan on his map of 1658. It consisted of a grid of 80 feet wide streets containing forty neighbourhoods, 285 yards by 200 yards in size. “Each formed a separate parish with frontages on four great streets.” A parish church and churchyard were at the centre of each neighbourhood, of which the internal streets were 24 feet wide (Reddaway, 1939). Newcourt’s plan included a huge central space, four parishes in size, which was to contain the Guildhall and markets. Each quarter of the city, comprising ten parishes, had a central square, with a new St Paul’s Cathedral occupying the square on the high land in the south-west quarter.

In planning Savannah, Georgia, in 1788, James Oglethorpe may well have had in mind the neighbourhood units that Cataneo had shown in his plan of 1567 (Bacon, 1967). It is perhaps more likely that Oglethorpe was aware of Newcourt’s plan of 1666, and would have seen Philadelphia growing according to the plan Thomas Holme prepared for William Penn in 1683. It is reasonable to assume that Philadelphia was the antecedent of William Light’s 1836 plan for Adelaide, and the idea of setting the city in parklands would come not only from Roebuck but also T.J. Maslen’s *The Friend of Australia,* published in 1830.

Philosophical Radicals of the Twentieth Century

In the second half of the nineteenth century the foundations were laid for what Patrick Geddes described as the "neotechnic era." In the early twentieth century, electricity, the telephone, the power station, the oil well, the motor car, the radio and many other inventions created a new Technology. Geddes widened the scope of planning and advocated bringing together in constructive citizenship the too long separated aspects of the conduct of life. He influenced the planning philosopher, Lewish Mumford, and the practising planners, Raymond Unwin and Patrick Abercrombie. (Geddes, 1915).

Ebenezer Howard, a contemporary of Geddes, synthesized many of the ideas and proposals put forward by the Philosophical Radicals and other nineteenth century reformers, and provided an important link between nineteenth and twentieth century planning in his book, *Tomorrow,* first published in 1898. Wakefield had shown the way to build new towns in the colonies, Howard was to promote the building of new towns in Britain. In 1901 he founded the Garden Cities Association (now the Town and Country Planning Association), and shortly afterwards published the third edition of his book *Garden Cities of Tomorrow*. In 1903 he was the main force in the establishment of first Garden City Limited, which was to build Letchworth Garden City.

In the postscript to his book (1902), Howard wrote that "the Garden City Association was very fortunate. It secured the services of Thomas Adams, a young Scotchman, who has proved active, energetic and resourceful – to whose suggestion was due the Conference held in September, 1901, at Mr Cadbury's beautiful village of Bournville, and the Conference held in July, 1902, at Messrs Lever's beautiful village of Port Sunlight, which have done more than anything else to make the Garden City Association and its project known to the great public, and to give our members ocular proof of the feasibility – indeed, the wonderful success – of undertakings in so many respects like our own" (Howard, 1902).

Colonel Light incorporated parklands in his plan for Adelaide (1836). Howard used the plan to illustrate "The true principle on which all towns should grow...The city is built up. How does it grow? It grows by leaping over the 'Park Lands' and establishing North Adelaide."

Welwyn, the second garden city to be promoted by Howard, was started by a limited dividend corporation in 1920. After the war it was a well established going concern, but following a political decision it was completed by one of the public corporations established under the New Towns Act, 1946. The application of the Town Planning Act, 1947, ensured that the land surrounding the New Towns remained agricultural.

(Sir) Frederic Osborn was the most influential disciple of Ebenezer Howard. Throughout his long life he was a very active member of the Town and Country Planning Association and for a long time Editor of the journal *Town and Country Planning*. His considerable planning knowledge was based on experience, starting at an early age in the office of a London housing society, and later as secretary/manager of the Howard Cottage Society in Letchworth, the First Garden City. Before leaving Letchworth in 1919 he advocated the building of new towns in his *New Towns after the War,* 1918, (reissued in 1942). From 1919 to 1936, he was Estate Manager, Welwyn Garden City, when Louis de Soissons and Arthur Kenyon were designing housing and site plans which were superior to all others of that period (de Soissons, Louis, and Kenyon, Arthur, 1927). Osborn was able to draw on this outstanding practical experience when he was the most knowledgeable and leading member of Lord Reith's *New Towns Committee* (Final Report of the New Towns Committee, July, 1946).

Ebenezer Howard's discovery of 1901, Thomas Adams, the first full time secretary of the Garden Cities Association, became an adviser to John Burns, the Minister who steered the first Housing and Town Planning Act through Parliament (1909). Adams was one of the nine distinguished founders of the (Royal) Town Planning Institute, and came to be a leader in town planning not only in Britain but also in Canada and the United States of

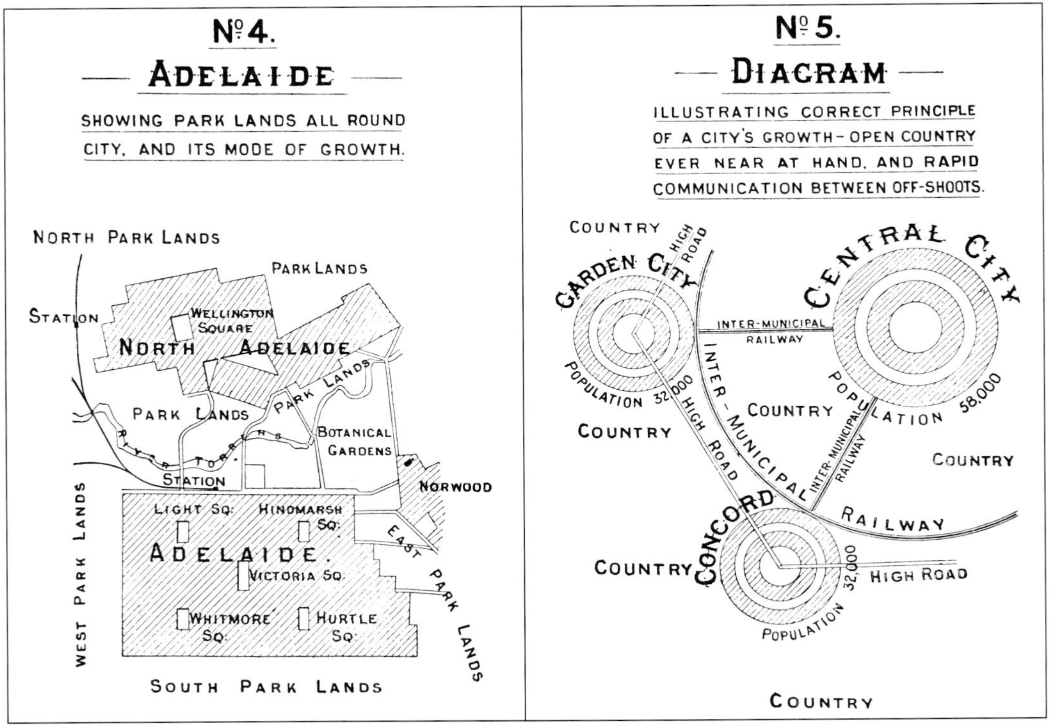

Two diagrams from Ebenezer Howard's GARDEN CITIES OF TOMORROW illustrating the principle of metropolitan growth as a constellation of cities.

America. He went to Canada in 1914 as Town Planning Adviser to the Commission on Conservation, producing model reports on rural and sociological conditions, land use and the resettlement of ex-servicemen. In 1920, he was largely responsible for the establishment of the Town Planning Institute of Canada, and even when working in the United States remained as consultant to the Canadian Government until 1930.

Adams proved to be an outstanding leader of a diverse professional team which produced the monumental *Regional Survey of New York and its Environs* for the Russell Sage Foundation. Published in New York in 1929, it may now best be known because of the sociologist, Clarence A. Perry's proposed plan for a school-centred neighbourhood unit, with through traffic roads on the perimeter.

Before returning to England in the early nineteen-thirties Thomas Adams taught at Harvard University and advised the Presidents of both Harvard and the Massachusetts Institute of Technology on the establishment of post-graduate courses in city planning. In his inimitable report to the Harvard President, he suggested that three classes of students should be admitted, namely, those concerned with (i) the science of enquiry, (ii) the art of creative design, and (iii) the system of administration. In 1950, the Schuster Committee reached a similar conclusion, and found that the University of Liverpool was establishing a master's degree course as if in response to their recommendations (Schuster, 1950). Frederick Adams put his father's report into effect at MIT in 1934. The University of Liverpool followed suit in 1950 when I was the Lever Professor of Civic Design.

Thomas Adams started his working life as a journalist in Dundee. His reports and books were written in plain, intelligent English. My wife was an assistant in his London office in the year before the Second World War. The word *jitterbug* was coming into use. He liked it. Pronouncing the word with a delightful Scottish burr, he told her "you may enrich the language but you must never pervert it."

Thomas Adams and Raymond Unwin died in 1940, the year in which London was being heavily bombed and the publication of the Barlow Royal Commission's Report marked a turning point in planning history. Adams, after spending most of his professional life in North America, died in East Sussex; Unwin, who had pioneered the development of town planning and housing in Britain, died in New York. Patrick Abercrombie (1879-1957), who had been the most influential member of the Barlow Royal Commission, was the inspiring leader of the small professional teams which produced the *County of London Plan, 1943,* and the *Greater London Plan, 1944.* For over thirty years, he had been learning from the philosophical radicals of the nineteenth and twentieth centuries, and went further than Unwin had been able to go.

Raymond Unwin started his professional life as an engineer but made his name as the most influential architect and planner in Britain from the turn of the century until 1936, when at the age of 73 he was appointed Visiting Professor at Columbia University. In 1896 he entered into partnership with his cousin, Barry Parker. Their first notable achievement was the design of New Earswick, near York, a model housing project, built for a Village Trust established by Joseph Rowntree (1836-1925) who, like Robert Owen at the beginning of the nineteenth century, was intent on improving the lot of his factory workers. Unwin remained in partnership with Parker until 1914, when he became chief architect and planner for the Ministry of Health, which was responsible for housing and planning. On his retirement from the civil service in 1928 he became Technical Adviser to the Greater London Regional Planning Committee, which in its Second Report of March 1933, provided some of the groundwork for Patrick Abercrombie's far more ambitious and comprehensive Greater London Plan, 1944 (Unwin, 1933).

Raymond Unwin became a member of the Fabian Society early in life, believing that "cooperation between men of different capacity is the secret of advanced power and progress." In 1904, he met (Dame) Henrietta Barnett, social scientist and wife of Canon Barnett, who founded Toynbee Hall in 1885. At the time of their meeting William Beveridge was a sub-warden of Toynbee Hall. During the Second World War in 1941, he was appointed

communities with a population of fifty thousand people would not merely be more adequately governed, probably, than one city that contained a million: it would, for example, give an opportunity for twenty mayors or city managers against one in the big center. This rule holds true in every other part of society...With our overgrown institutions, overgrown colleges, overgrown corporations, overgrown cities, is it any wonder that we easily become the victims of propaganda machines, routineers and dictators?" (Mumford, 1938).

As early as 1926, ideas developed by the small group of friends who had formed the Regional Planning Association of America were put into effect in the now almost forgotten Basic Plan for the future growth of New York (Stein, Wright, 1926). The principles underlying the plan may be compared with the Greater London Plan, 1944, and the Strategy Plan for Canberra, 1969, generally known as the Y-Plan. All three proposed that outward, urban growth should be in a constellation of new towns.

Lewis Mumford compared the eighty-two page Report prepared for the State of New York by Henry Wright with the seven volume report on the Metropolitan District of New York, prepared under the chairmanship of Thomas Adams (Adams, 1929). "Wright's report dealt not only with past facts but with new social and economic emergents: as a result the work of Wright and his associates laid a foundation for the regional planning movement throughout the United States. the Russell Sage report, on the other hand, was obsolete even at the moment of its original formulation, to say nothing of its final summary: a compendious handbook on how not to approach the future, and of what not to do. Adams' report committed the city to a continuance of its past mistakes: Henry Wright's report showed, in the existing situation, the latent possibilities for a new order: not a passive contribution but a re-integration."

"Do not ignore the difference between these two orders of thinking – it underlies the approach to the whole problem of urban re-settlement and rebuilding that now confronts the Western World."

“The problem has two sides to it: one is the building up of new centers great and small, cutting out morbid tissue, restoring functional relationships that have lapsed, giving them, in the process of renewal, a parity with the newer communities” (Mumford, 1938).

Influence now flowed both ways across the Atlantic, as Mumford’s books reached a wide audience in Britain and reinforced the social and urban philosophy to which the planners of the Town and Country Planning Association could appeal. The popular and political support for their ideas was at its peak when the disasters of depression and war created their greatest opportunities.

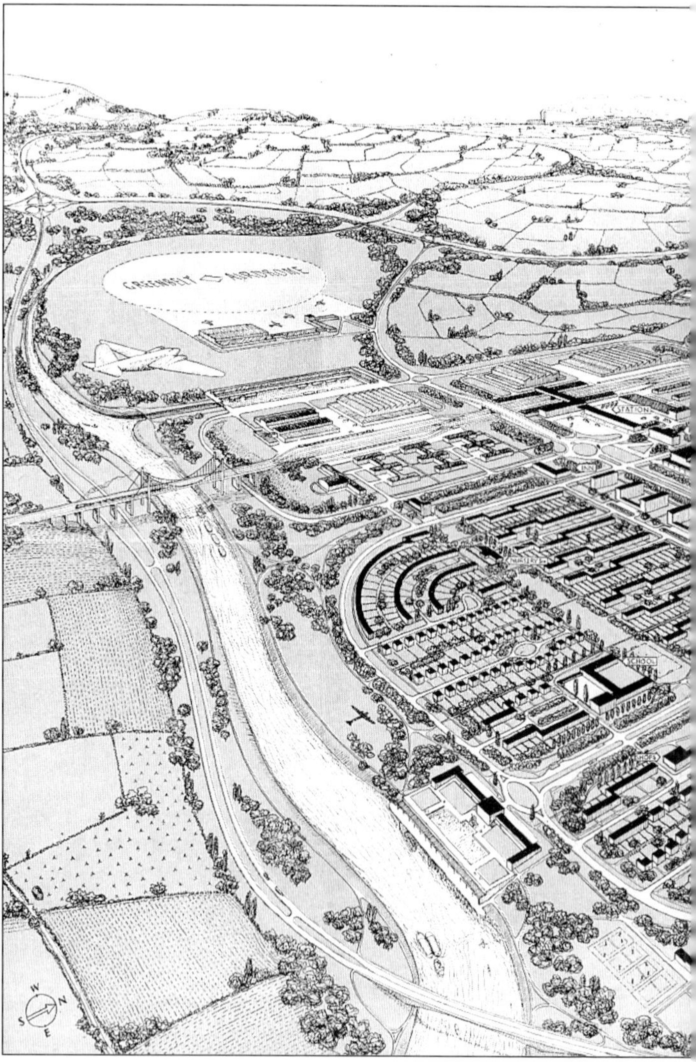

A bird's eye view of a hypothetical NEW TOWN showing its relationship to the parent
the Second World War. Published in October, 1942, by *Pictorial Education Q*

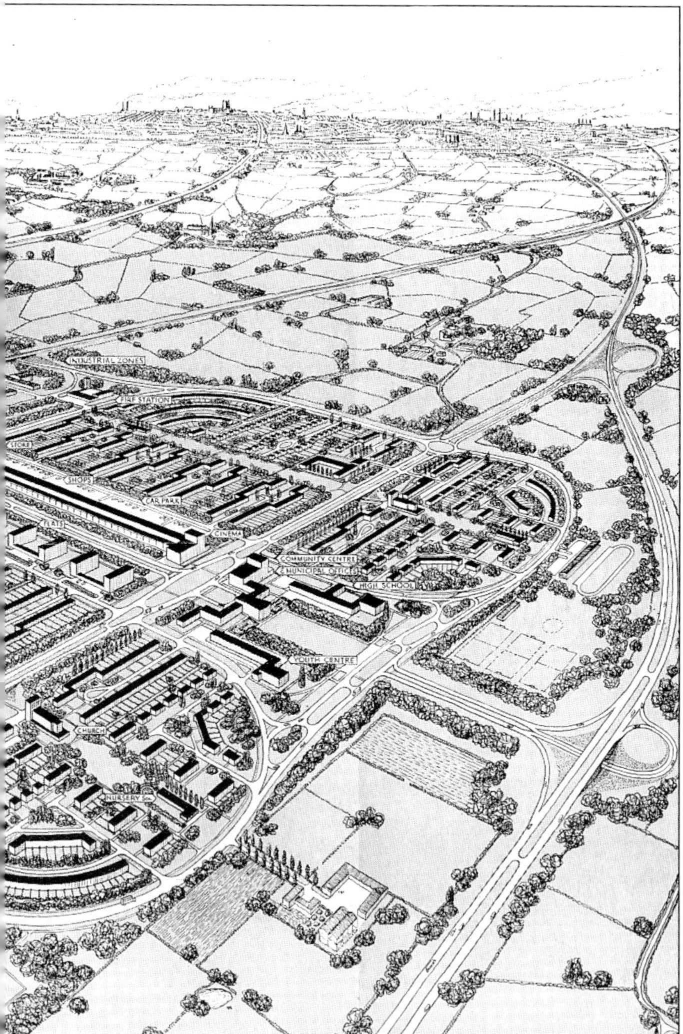

A NEW TOWN

y and the countryside. Designed and drawn by Gordon Stephenson in the middle of
terly, as a wall sheet printed in colour to be exhibited in Secondary Schools.

National Leadership in Depression and War

In August 1941, four months before the Japanese attack on Pearl Harbour brought the United States into the Second World War, Winston Churchill, Prime Minister of the United Kingdom, and Franklin D. Roosevelt, President of the United States, met on a battleship off the coast of Canada. In their ATLANTIC CHARTER they outlined a broad picture of the world as they wanted it. It is worth recalling the eight points of that charter over half a century later, in a world which seems to have lost some of that simple idealism, and confidence in the capacities of democratic government. They said:

First, their countries seek no aggrandisement, territorial or other.

Second, they desire to see no territorial changes that do not accord with the freely expressed wishes of the peoples concerned.

Third, they respect the right of all peoples to choose the form of government under which they will live; and they wish to see sovereign rights and self-government restored to those who have been forcibly deprived of them.

Fourth, they will endeavour, with due respect for their existing obligations, to further enjoyment by all States, great or small, victor or vanquished, of access, on equal terms, to the trade and to the raw materials of the world which are needed for their economic prosperity.

Fifth, they desire to bring about the greatest collaboration between all nations in the economic field, with the object of securing, for all, improved labour standards, economic advancement and social security.

Sixth, after the final destruction of Nazi tyranny, they hope to see established a peace which will afford to all nations the means of dwelling in safety within their own boundaries and which will afford assurance that all men in all the lands may live out their lives in freedom from fear and want.

Seventh, such a peace should enable all men to traverse the high seas and oceans without hindrance.

Eighth, they believe all of the nations of the world, for realistic as well as spiritual reasons, must come to the abandonment of the use of force. Since no future peace can be maintained if land, sea, or air armaments continue to be employed by nations which threaten, or may threaten aggression outside of their frontiers, they believe, pending the establishment of a wider and permanent system of general security, that the disarmament of such nations is essential. They will likewise aid and encourage all other practical measures which will lighten for peace-loving peoples the crushing burden of armament.

It is likely that the Atlantic Charter was drafted by Harry Hopkins, Roosevelt's closest adviser during his four terms as President. Under the Roosevelt Administration a great effort had been made to lift the United States out of the world depression of the 1930s. To overcome mass unemployment the Government adopted the Keynesian strategy of initiating a vast series of "works" projects. Instead of "doles" the Government provided work on useful schemes. These included the building of 44,000 miles of highways, 19,000 bridges, 1,500 schools, 2,000 parks and playgrounds, and public buildings of all kinds in all communities. Many thousands of dwellings were improved, theatrical productions were organised, and there were projects for writers, artists and technicians. In 1938 there were 3,474,000 persons employed on "works projects." The American concept of post-war planning was greatly influenced by this experience. By 1942, the National Resources Planning Board had built up a reservoir of planned projects which could be executed as labour became available in the post-war years.

The National Resources Planning Board defined a series of planning objectives in a Report which the President transmitted to the Congress. The Report said that "any new declaration of personal rights, any translation of freedom in modern terms applicable to the people of the United States here and now must include:

1. The right to work, usefully and creatively, through the productive years.

development and, where necessary, should be given opportunity for dealing with the problem on a regional rather than a municipal basis. In cases approved by the Central Authority, financial assistance should be available from Government funds.

The powers of the Central Authority should also include:

(a) Collection and co-ordination of information relating to location of industry, now in the possession of the various Government Departments.

(b) Research: and collection of information as to the national resources – land, agriculture, amenities, etc. – that may be affected by industrial location.

(c) Advice to Government, local authorities and industrialists as to problems of location.

The Barlow Royal Commission unanimously recommended the Government appoint a body of experts to examine the question of compensation, betterment and development generally.

In a minority report, three members of the Commission, namely, Patrick Abercrombie, Herbert Elvin and Mrs Hermione Hichens strongly made a case for a new Ministry of Planning.

Wartime Initiatives

In 1940, shortly after the bombing of London and other British cities began, Churchill asked Lord Reith, the newly appointed Minister of Works and Buildings, to form a small Reconstruction Group to concern itself with the rebuilding of war damaged areas and post-war town planning. In the same year Reith had previously been Minister of Information and Minister of Transport. His relations with the Prime Minister were probably uneasy. It was rumoured in civil service circles that Churchill referred to Lord Reith, a tall austere man, as "old Wuthering Heights". Before he left his Ministerial post to accept a commission in the Royal Navy, Reith had firmly established a small Reconstruction Group. Its members were H. Chalton Bradshaw, William Holford, John Dower, Thomas Sharp and myself. It was organized and led by Harold Graham Vincent, an experienced public servant, who gradually increased its membership. With the Barlow Report as his guide, Vincent persuaded Reith to commission what became the Scott report on country planning, and the Uthwatt report on planning problems of compensation and betterment.

In 1941 Churchill appointed William Beveridge as Chairman of an Interdepartmental Committee on Social Insurance and Allied services. The Beveridge Report – the blue-print for the post-war welfare state – appeared in the following year.

In response to the Barlow, Beveridge, Scott and Uthwatt reports, the coalition government established the Ministry of Town and Country Planning in 1943, and the Ministry of National Insurance in 1944. The succeeding Attlee government extended and strengthened the powers of the Ministry of Health, the Board of Trade and the Ministry of Agriculture and Fisheries. The first Minister of Town and Country Planning, William Shepherd Morrison (1943-45) presided over a department formed by an amalgamation of the Reconstruction Group and those in the Ministry of Health who had administered pre-war town and country planning. Morrison was succeeded by Lewis Silkin

(1945-50) who was responsible for the New Towns Act of 1946 and the Town and Country Planning Act of 1947, and implemented policies which, in particular, ensured the building of new towns, the planned re-development of bomb-damaged areas, and the provision of land for housing.

Another Reith initiative had prompted the London County Council to commission the first of two London plans which proved to be landmarks in planning history, namely, the *County of London Plan*, 1943, (Forshaw, J.H. and Abercrombie, Patrick, 1943). the new Ministry commissioned the complementary *Greater London Plan* (1944), also by Patrick Abercrombie. Those bold plans were whole-heartedly accepted by a compassionate people who had suffered badly from aerial bombardment. Under the frontispiece of the County of London Plan there is a quotation from a speech the Prime Minister made in the House of Commons in October, 1940. It reads "Most painful is the number of small houses inhabited by working folk which has been destroyed…We will rebuild them, more to our credit than some of them were before. London, Liverpool, Manchester, Birmingham may have much more to suffer, but they will rise from their ruins, more healthy and, I hope, more beautiful…In all my life I have never been treated with so much kindness as by the people who have suffered most."

Much of the credit for establishing the new planning institutions belonged to H.G. Vincent, who led Lord Reith's Reconstruction Group. He graduated from Cambridge University in 1914 with a First Class Mathematical Tripos and was in the British Army in Europe during the First World War. In 1919 he entered the Treasury, and for nine years from 1928 to 1936 he was Private Secretary to successive Prime Ministers. As a result he had an excellent understanding of what could be done in the parliament and civil service. In 1936 he was appointed as a Principal Assistant Secretary to the Committee of Imperial Defence, and in 1939 was transferred to the Ministry of Food under Lord Woolton. It was said that Vincent played a key role in devising the very successful British food rationing system. Next year he moved to lead Lord Reith's Reconstruction Group. There he took up many recommendations of the Barlow Royal Commission. The Scott and Uthwatt Committees were established, and reported in 1942. By 1943 Vincent's main aim was achieved with the creation of the Ministry of Town and Country Planning. He had worked wonders, but in the new Ministry he remained a Principal Assistant Secretary under higher-ranked civil servants. After four eventful years his initiating role was over. He then spent five years in the Ministries of Production and Aviation, was knighted in 1953, and retired in 1956 after seven years in the uncreative position of Secretary, Government Hospitality.

Until 1943 Vincent had been the driving force in the group concerned with postwar planning. When the Ministry of Town and Country Planning was formed, the group was amalgamated with the planning division of the Ministry of Health, and Evelyn Sharp became Deputy Secretary. From the time of her arrival she was the dominant administrative decision maker. In 1955, she became Permanent Secretary of the all-embracing Ministry of Housing and Local Government. But it was the wartime initiatives which bore fruit in the reports and plans which established the institutions and directions of planning for decades ahead.

The Scott Report

The Barlow report concerned only the towns and the industrial population. To examine what the Barlow Commission had not been able to study, Lord Reith appointed a Committee, with Lord Justice Scott as chairman, to consider the country and the rural population. At the time more than 80 percent of the land of England and Wales was in agricultural use, and less than 20 per cent of the population lived and worked in rural areas. If industry was running alternately downhill and uphill between the wars, declining in one place and spreading in another, agriculture was generally on the decline.

The Scott Committee reported in August, 1942, (Scott, 1942). The conclusions of the Committee were based on the assumption that Government policy would include the maintenance of a prosperous and progressive agriculture. The Committee stated that "it is our firm belief that a vital incentive to the war effort is the presentation of a clear picture of a better world which lies ahead and which, if plans are drawn up and the essential preparations made in advance, can be achieved after this struggle is over. To delay planning and the legislation to carry the plans into effect until the time for action is upon us – the end of the war – we believe to be a fatal error."

The main recommendations of the Scott Committee follow:

A big rural housing programme should be undertaken.

Low cost electricity should be made available throughout the country.

Special consideration should be given to the provision of a main water supply to all towns and villages, farms, market gardens and allotments.

Steps should be taken to provide social centres in all villages.

Every village should be provided with playing fields.

Afforestation should be extended on poor land. National forest parks should be established.

Local Authorities should supervise and maintain footpaths. "Hikers' highways" should be recognised, and a right of way for walks provided around the whole coast line.

The establishment of a national parks scheme, including the coast of England and Wales, is long overdue.

With the extension of holidays with pay, further holiday camps should be provided.

Where land is defaced in the process of extracting minerals, responsibility for restoring the surface should rest primarily on those working the minerals.

The disposal and future use of war factories established in the countryside should be determined by the Central Planning Authority.

Before new towns are established in country areas, vacant or derelict industrial sites in existing towns should be fully utilised but introduction of carefully regulated industry into the towns of country areas would be beneficial.

Tracts of good soil near towns and villages should be kept for open spaces and market gardens and allotments. Allotment holders should have security of tenure.

All new villages and country towns should be near but not on main traffic roads, and all existing villages and country towns on main traffic routes should be by-passed.

New buildings in country areas should use to the full all the possibilities which new materials and new building techniques have made available.

Bold planning of new trunk highways is needed, rather than the continuance of piecemeal widening of existing roads.

Railways should come under planning control. Railway level crossings on important roads should be eliminated, and many old railway bridges should be rebuilt.

Control should be exercised over the siting and character of advertisements.

All land should be planned nationally and locally.

The Scott Report complemented the Barlow Report. Nearly all the recommendations were put into effect, resulting in security for agriculture in the post war years, and a seemly countryside attractive to residents, visitors and tourists alike. The Report was written by Thomas Sharp, a planning innovator and writer of distinction. While the Committee was in session, I shared a room with Thomas Sharp, enjoyed his knowledge and company and learned to respect his professional probity. The latter was very evident in his occasional altercations with Dudley Stamp, the geographer Vice-Chairman of the Committee. Lord Justice Scott was aged and slow-moving. Dudley Stamp was quick witted and knowledgeable, having before the war undertaken a monumental Land Utilisation Survey of the whole country. Stamp was ambitious and, as Consultant to the Ministry of Agriculture after the war, had a good deal to say about the future use of agricultural land. He probably had this in view when, against the Committee's findings, he wanted the Ministry of Agriculture to have the power to veto urban development even where it was seemingly inevitable. Sharp was a stickler for recording exactly the decisions of the Committee. In comparison, Stamp was biased.

Among Sharp's many books the *Anatomy of the Village* (1946) may be the best known. It examined the social as well as the physical characteristics of English villages, and showed how they might be planned in future. Sharp designed four new villages in Northumberland for the Forestry Commission and a seaside village in South Wales.

The Uthwatt Report

The Report of the Uthwatt Committee was published in the month following the publication of the Scott Committee. Following the recommendation of the Barlow Royal Commission, Lord Reith appointed an expert committee under the chairmanship of Mr Justice Uthwatt to consider problems of compensation and betterment resulting from physical planning (Uthwatt, 1942). The background to the Uthwatt recommendations was to be found in the introductory statement in the Report:

"The first assumption we have made is that national planning is intended to be a reality and a permanent feature of the administration of the internal affairs of this country. We assume that it will be directed to ensuring that the best use is made of land with a view to securing economic efficiency for the community and well being for the individual, and that it will be recognised that this involves the subordination to the public good of the personal interests and wishes of landowners. Unreserved acceptance of this conception of planning is vital to a successful reconstruction policy, for every aspect of a nation's activity is ultimately dependent on land. The denser the population, the more intensive the use of land becomes in order that the limited area may be capable of furnishing the services required; the more complex the productive organisation of society, the more highly developed must be the control of land utilisation exercised by or on behalf of the community."

Among the recommendations of the Uthwatt Committee were the following:

(i) Amendments to the law of town planning so as to extend and simplify the power of acquisition of land for large-scale development and to modify rules for assessment of compensation.

(ii) The acquisition by the State of "development rights" in all land outside built up areas; compensation to be paid on March,

1939, values for these "development rights", which would be considered as a whole and not piecemeal.

(iii) A levy of a tax of 75 per cent, on increase in land value not due to the enterprise of the owner and not including agricultural land.

The nationalisation of all development rights in undeveloped land was, essentially, built into the Town and Country Planning Act, 1947. It meant that no development could take place without the permission of the local planning authority. If permission were refused, except in special cases, no compensation would be paid. If granted, the increase in land value was to be subject to a development charge. In practice assessing development charges led to endless wrangling, sometimes akin to bargaining in an oriental market. Valuers in the new bureaucracy always seemed to differ from valuers in private practice. The chequered system was altered in 1954, dismantled in 1959, revived with the Land Commission in 1966, and finally abandoned in 1970. A solution to the problem of compensation and betterment has yet to be found. The nationalisation of development rights in undeveloped land has not been challenged.

The London Plans

The County of London Plan (1943) and the Greater London Plan (1944) set new standards for post-war planning. They assisted "the Ministry in considering the methods and machinery for the reconstruction of Town and Country." They provided background knowledge and material for the preparation of planning legislation and, in particular, the New Towns Act (1946) and the Town and Country Planning Act (1947).

At that time Patrick Abercrombie was the only person in Britain, and perhaps the world, who could successfully have led the County of London and the Greater London planning teams. For over thirty years he had been extending his range of knowledge and experience beyond that of any other planner in Europe or North America. He and John Forshaw, Architect to the London County Council, were the authors of the County of London Plan, 1943. The County Council provided a staff of 46, of whom the majority were professional planners or architects. Wesley Dougill, who had been Abercrombie's Senior Lecturer in the University of Liverpool Department of Civic Design, was introduced to manage the planning group and died, probably through overwork, before the report was completed. He, Bellamy, Ling, Mackenzie, Macfarlane, Marshall and Richards undertook original research.

Putting together the Greater London team was more difficult. By 1942 professional planners were hard to find. The Ministry of Town and Country Planning paid Abercrombie the princely sum of 3,000 guineas, and found and paid his team, which completed the work in about eighteen months. There were seven professional members, of whom five had started their careers as architects. Harry Stewart was, in effect office manager. An Inspector in the Ministry of Health, he had acted as Chairman of the Technical Committee of the Standing Conference on London Regional Planning, which had been dormant since 1936. Of the other six, three came from the London County Council team and continued with the work they had begun on the County of London Plan, namely, Macfarlane on Industry, Richards on Communications, and Prasad acting as a general purpose member. Of the other three, Tom Coote was the most experienced, having worked between the wars for Adshead, Davidge and the Essex County Council. He had started his professional life as a surveyor. His knowledge of the London region was, without exaggeration, encyclopaedic. He commanded Abercrombie's great respect.

Peter Shepheard graduated in Architecture in the University of Liverpool in 1936, and the year after that was Lever Research Fellow in the Department of Civic Design. At the beginning of the war he joined an engineer to work on the design of a large explosives factory and came straight from that job to the Greater London team. Shepheard was a brilliant draftsman, took charge of the illustrations, and worked with me on the detailed studies in Chapter 11 (Greater London Plan, 1944). He and Coote later joined me in the Ministry's Planning Technique Section of the Research Division. After the war Shepheard was a partner in an architectural practice and, in turn, became President of the Landscape Institute and the Royal Institute of British Architects, and Dean of the Faculty of Architecture and Planning in the University of Pennsylvania. My position was unusual. In the Ministry my job was to develop the Planning Technique Section, and in this capacity I acted as liaison officer with the London County Council planning team. Later, Abercrombie and the Permanent Secretary reached an agreement that I should work part-time with the Greater London team and act as a link with the Ministry. This meant that the knowledge we were building up in Planning Technique could immediately be applied, and in practice amplified.

There are two good examples of the two-way transfer of knowledge. *Chapter 8* of the *Greater London Plan,* concerned with community planning standards, resulted from the work of one of the several wartime interdepartmental committees dealing with reconstruction. The principal contributors were Henry Jenkins, an Assistant Secretary in the Ministry of Education, Judith Ledeboer, an Architect in the Ministry of Health in the role that Unwin had played in the First World War, and myself, representing the Ministry of Town and Country Planning. Chapter 8 drew on technical exercises we undertook in the Ministry's Planning Technique Section, and gave dimensions to the ideas about community and neighbourhood planning expressed very clearly by Howard, Geddes and Mumford. It also set standards for a new school system and playing fields proposed by the Minister of Education, R.A. Butler, and new housing standards later published in the Housing Manual by the Ministry of Health. I wrote Chapter 8, and Chapter 11 resulted from detailed studies made by Peter Shepheard, Tom Coote and myself. T.E. North, the Borough Architect and Planning Officer of West Ham, supplied information and ideas for a redevelopment scheme for three badly damaged neighbourhoods in West Ham. The illustration of a redevelopment scheme for two neighbourhoods, each of 8000 population (*Greater London Plan,* 1944, Chapter 11) is strikingly similar to a contemporary proposal to demolish an area of tower blocks and replace them with low-rise terraces.

Looking back, it is hard to believe that the Greater London Plan was produced at breakneck speed. By today's standards the professional team was ridiculously small, and was forced to move from office to office four times, twice through bomb damage. The drafting team was makeshift, and never more than seven in number – six women, and an Irish architect who hardly ever put in a good day's work. Abercrombie, incredible man, ignored difficulties. Coote, Shepheard and I were a supporting inner cabinet. We shared all our thoughts and took no notice of the clock.

I first heard Abercrombie lecture in 1928 and was completely captivated from then onwards. Returning to Liverpool in 1932, after two years in Paris, I was fortunate to be recalled by Charles Reilly to be a Lecturer and Studio Instructor in the School of Architecture, and for the next four years sat in on most of Abercrombie's lectures. He hardly ever repeated himself and was constantly referring to his consulting work. The combination of teaching and practice is essential if a student is to learn how to cope with the real world of architecture and planning. Abercrombie gladly accepted my proposal to design a theoretical city for a master's degree. It was to emulate Tony Garnier's *Ville Industrielle.* Surprisingly he was enthusiastic, but I got more and more overloaded in my spare time as the secretary of a committee helping to get teachers, social democrats, trade unionists, communists, Jews and professional people out of Nazi Germany. The Greater London Plan and its aftermath gave me the opportunity to help lay the planning foundation of a fair number of new towns.

Raymond Unwin had worked on a Greater London plan during a sad period in the world's history, with mass unemployment in Europe and North America and Hitler in the ascendancy. Abercrombie's Greater London Plan was prepared when bombs were still falling, but the successful outcome of the war was only a matter of time. London was full of American soldiers and airmen and everyone was full of hope. Unwin had been enmeshed in a committee system, working with the Technical Committee of the Standing Conference on London Regional Planning. The Standing Conference had been standing still from the early days of the Great Depression, when Unwin's Second Report signalled the end of what was virtually a one man show (Unwin, 1933). By contrast, Abercrombie was as free as a bird, responsible in theory to a committee of local government officers, but in fact only to the Minister. Abercrombie was able to start from where Unwin had finished. This was particularly so in regard to three main elements: the highway system, housing, and the concept of the Green Belt. In Unwin's time, the only way to establish a greenbelt was to acquire the land. This The London County Council had started to do in 1936.

The 1947 Act altered all that, and signalled the end of a forty year struggle to establish planning and the planning profession. By the end of the Second World War there were some 1,700 members of the Royal Town Planning Institute; now there are more than ten times that number. Therein lies the rub. Most modern day planners spend endless time on committees, study groups and working parties, and fill numerous files. It is impossible to imagine an Abercrombie emerging from a world buried under paper. Yet we need new Abercrombies if only to interpret the will of modern society and give it a sense of direction. Abercrombie was at home with all kinds of people, was a good listener, had started life as an architect, and was both intelligent and creative. He practised what Geddes and Mumford had preached.

Low and High Housing

In keeping with Churchill's 1940 promise, peace brought a great burst of housing construction and reconstruction.

After the First World War, the provision of affordable housing became a main government objective. During the 1920s many housing estates were developed by local authorities, with Treasury assistance. In the 1930s the emphasis was on slum clearance. Walk-up tenements were built which were not only more costly but also unsatisfactory for families with children.

After the Second World War, the immediate building priorities were affordable housing, factories and schools. Once more, local authorities were to be the main housing providers. Where possible, war damaged houses were restored or rebuilt, temporary prefabricated houses were built on cleared areas and the edges of parks, and permanent houses were built on suburban fringes, and later in new towns. Beset by the need to be economically stringent, the Attlee Government financed 200,000 dwellings per year.

At a planning conference in Southport in 1951, shortly before a general election and at Lord Woolton's instigation, Harold Macmillan promised that a second Churchill Government would finance 300,000 dwellings per year. More than anything else, this helped to win the election. As Minister of Housing and Local Government Macmillan achieved the target he had set.

The achievement had some social costs. The Government did not allow the London County Council to provide housing in the New Towns. As a consequence, the Council sought land in the

Green Belt or in low density sections of the built area. It acquired about 100 acres in Roehampton, on the edge of Richmond Park, where the density prescribed by the Greater London Plan was to be 100 persons per acre, with terrace houses intended for families with children. Instead the design was dominated by heavily subsidised flats in widely spaced towers and high rise slabs. Built between 1952 and 1956, it was aclaimed in the architectural press, and set an example for other local authorities. Compared with terrace houses, high rise flats were extravagantly subsidised, despite being unsuitable for families with children. In a number of cities, many have been demolished or refurbished for higher income groups.

Philosophical Radicals of the Second World War

Harold Vincent, Patrick Abercrombie and other public servants, planners and architects deserve great credit for their contributions to the development of effective and compassionate planning. But they could have achieved little without broad national encouragement and powerful political leadership. The new Ministry of Town and Country Planning was formed when winning the war was only a matter of time, with the Soviet Union and the United States of America fully engaged. The parliament, the civil service, the fighting services and the country as a whole were determined that the lesson of wartime planning would forever remove the kind of laissez-faire which had led to the Great Depression and the advent of Mussolini, Hitler and a Japan seeking to dominate Asia by military conquest. Fortunately there were philosophical radicals of great courage and resolve in the War Cabinet. Among the most remarkable were Winston Churchill, Clement Attlee and Lord Woolton.

In the English speaking world, Churchill and Roosevelt were towering figures. Both introduced into government men and women who were destined to change attitudes and actions during and after the war. In the public mind, Churchill is remembered as an inspiring, defiant wartime leader, Roosevelt as a great social reformer who led America out of the Great Depression and to wartime victory. "The Churchill who helped to change the domestic face of Britain is usually neglected."

Churchill joined the British Army in 1895, and in the next five years served in Cuba, Pakistan, Egypt, the Sudan and Africa. From 1900-1906 he was Conservative Member of Parliament for Oldham, and from 1906-1908 Liberal Member for N.W. Manchester, serving as Under-Secretary of State for the Colonies. He then became the Conservative MP for Dundee, from 1908-1922, and in turn President of the Board of Trade, Home Secretary, First Lord of the Admiralty, Chancellor of the Duchy of Lancaster, Minister for Munitions, Secretary of State for War, for Air and for the Colonies. From 1924-1929, he was an innovative

Chancellor of the Exchequer, and then spent the next ten years out of Government but in Parliament, sometimes as a lone voice, speaking against Hitler and all that he stood for. With the Second World War fast approaching, he was recalled by Neville Chamberlain as First Lord of the Admiralty, and early in 1940 became Prime Minister.

Writing in the *Guardian Weekly* (17 January 1993) Martin Gilbert shows quite clearly that Churchill's role as a politician was as important as that of the wartime leader.

"As early as 1897, Churchill, then a very young Conservative, was speaking publicly in favour of making workmen shareholders in the profits of the enterprises for which they worked. He was a pioneer in the establishment of compulsory arbitration procedures to allow industrial disputes to be given a neutral and fair hearing. He fought, in his Shops Bill, for drastically improved conditions on the shop-floor (with the House of Commons rejecting the most radical of his proposals). He introduced the principle and practice of compulsory breaks for meals in the workplace, and stressed that the march of industrial democracy was not only towards shorter hours of work, but also greater opportunities for leisure."

"During the coal dispute in 1926, Churchill tried over several months to persuade the Conservative cabinet to accept the basic principle of the minimum wage, and fought hard against the undercutting of miners' wages in areas of high unemployment. He believed that the state had substantial responsibilities towards the underprivileged and unfortunate, and, as Chancellor of the Exchequer, he introduced state pensions for widows and orphans. He was a leading advocate of a stiff tax on war profits after both world wars. He wanted to extend the age of compulsory education, and even more important, to make education and not class the basis for advancement. In 1940, he overruled the Admiralty examiners when they refused to give a naval cadetship to a man with a cockney accent."

"Churchill's wartime broadcasts are recalled as fire and brimstone against Germany. But in a broadcast in 1942 he called for a National Health Service based on broad and solid foundations."

"In this same broadcast he advocated compulsory national insurance 'from cradle to grave', and with educational opportunities extended, and fair competition for job selection so arranged, that Britain would draw its leaders 'from every kind of school and wearing every type of tie.' His concern that opportunity should be more widely based and that government should intervene to ensure a fairer society was constantly pressed on his cabinet."

As early as 1941, after the Battle of Britain, Churchill had appointed the Beveridge, Scott and Uthwatt committees to their tasks. In 1942 Clement Attlee became Deputy Prime Minister and in 1943 Lord Woolton became Minister of Reconstruction and Member of the War Cabinet. Attlee, as Prime Minister from 1945-51, was responsible for putting the largely agreed postwar reconstruction legislation into effect. Churchill succeeded him as Prime Minister in 1951, and resigned in 1955 at the age of 81. He had been a Member of Parliament from the beginning of the century, was honoured in every conceivable way, but despite his ancestry chose never to leave the House of Commons. He was a great parliamentarian who, even in the abysmal periods of the war, made important public announcements only in the House of Commons.

In 1955, the year in which Churchill resigned, Attlee was created an Earl. Churchill had graduated from Sandhurst Military College and started his career as a soldier. Attlee, who was nine years younger than Churchill, and an Oxford graduate, was called to the Bar and practised law from 1906-1908. During this time he joined the Fabian Society, the Independent Labour Party and the National Union of Clerks. In 1910 he spent the year as Secretary of Toynbee Hall, the University Settlement in Stepney. In the same year, Lord Woolton, then F.J. Marquis, was the Warden of the Liverpool University Settlement. It is worth noting that Beveridge was Sub-warden of Toynbee Hall, from 1903-1906, during Canon Barnett's reign as Warden, and at the time when Hampstead Garden Suburb was being built at the instigation of Mrs Barnett. It is therefore likely that Attlee would have met Raymond Unwin, a fellow Fabian.

Attlee left Toynbee Hall to lecture for a year in Ruskin College, and in 1913 was appointed Tutor and Lecturer in Social Science at the London School of Economics, a position he held until 1923. During the First World War he served in Europe and the Middle East, and was commissioned as a major in 1917. During his early years in politics he was always referred to as Major Attlee. He was elected Labour Mayor of Stepney immediately after the war, and in 1920 entered the House of Commons as Labour member for the Limehouse Division of Stepney, part of the working class docklands which were badly damaged during the numerous bombing raids on London. Stepney was one of the Reconstruction Areas studied in the County of London Plan, 1943.

In the War Cabinet, Attlee was, in turn, Lord Privy Seal, Secretary of State for Dominion Affairs, Lord President of the Council, and from 1942-45 Deputy Prime Minister. He succeeded Churchill as Prime Minister in 1945, and during the next six years was able to put into effect social and economic reconstruction conclusions reached by the Coalition Cabinet. Lewis Silkin, who had been Chairman of the London County Council Planning Committee during the war, succeeded W.S. Morrison as Minister of Town and Country Planning, and benefited from the wartime spade work of his predecessor. Silkin moved quickly in the final preparation of the New Towns Bill of 1946, and the Town and Country Planning Bill of 1947. As is the wont in politics, he got all the credit when they were enacted. The honours, should, perhaps, have been shared with Morrison and Churchill's remarkable wartime cabinet.

Churchill was an heroic figure who liked to be seen in an unusual hat and smoking a long Havana cigar. In 1941, he addressed the Canadian Parliament in Ottawa, where Yousuf Karsh photographed him and wrote "He was more than the great man of the twentieth century: he was even more than an institution. He has become and will always remain, a gigantic passage in human history" (Karsh, 1959).

In Churchill's shadow during the war, Attlee was a key figure in the coalition cabinet and a successful Prime Minister in the post-war reconstruction period. He was modest in appearance

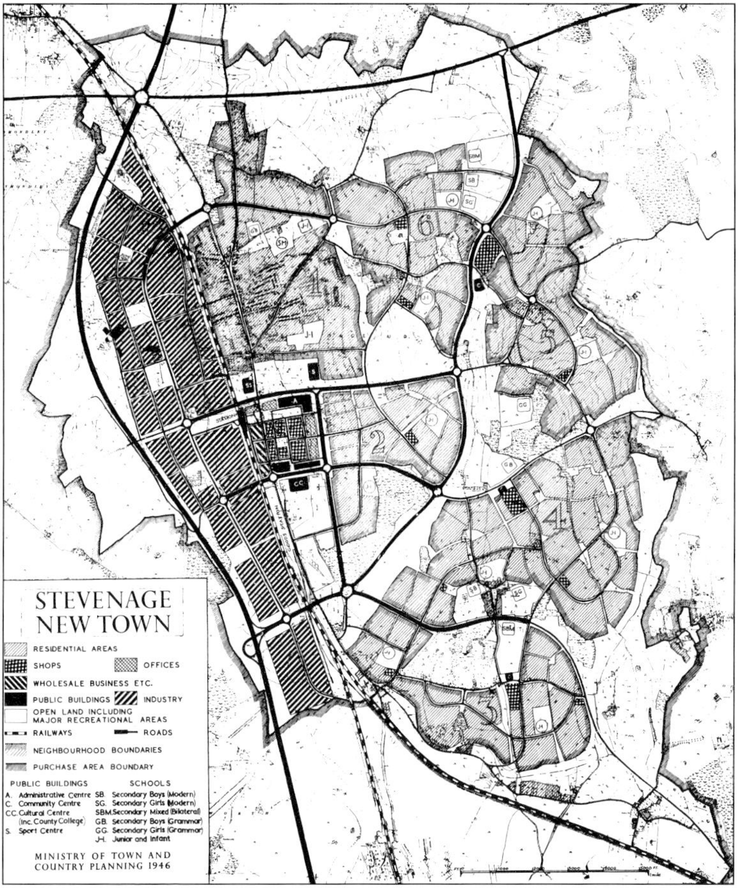

Stevenage was one of the eight new towns proposed in the Greater London Plan, 1944. The plan was prepared in the Ministry of Town and Country Planning before Parliament passed the New Towns Act, and was to be the prototype for the New Towns programme. Completed in June, 1946, the plan was accompanied by a 60 page report, a copy of which is now in the University of Liverpool Archives. The planning team was G. Stephenson, R.T. Kennedy, T.C. Coote, P.F. Shepheard and E.C. Claxton.

and demeanour, would be a perfect chairman, and when Prime Minister, as a guest of the Royal Institute of British Architects, proved himself to be an erudite and witty after-dinner speaker, without using notes. During his six years in 10 Downing Street, he could be seen, early in most mornings, walking with his dog in St James's Park, with no minders or security men in sight.

Unlike Churchill and Attlee, Lord Woolton was a successful business man, who was pressed into service at the beginning of the war as Director-General of Equipment and Stores in the Ministry of Supply. With Churchill as Prime Minister, he was appointed Minister of Food, 1940-43, and Minister of Reconstruction, 1943-45. During and after the life of the Attlee Government, he was Chairman of the Conservative and Unionist Central Office, and in this role planned the advent of the second Churchill Government, 1951-55, in which he was Lord President of the Council.

Lord Woolton, then Frederick James Marquis, graduated from Manchester University, and for a time was Research Fellow in Economics before becoming Warden of the Liverpool University Settlement. From his early years he was an active Unitarian and interested in town planning. Patrick Abercrombie, who also came to Liverpool from Manchester, knew this, when, late in 1909, he invited him to write an article for the first number of the first volume of the *Town Planning Review.* Marquis echoed Geddes v. the City Beautiful Movement when he wrote "to summarise: town planning must become a conscious and thorough effort to direct and control the growth of cities, and of the outskirts of cities. It must aim at forcing upward the standard of life, class by class, securing for each the fullest possible exercise of freedom, but curbing always such individual initiative as would seem likely to trespass on the rights and liberties of others. Town planning postulates town comprehension; survey and conscious direction of forces must precede civic design. So we seem to be on the threshold of the period when the science of civics will direct the development of towns, and will collate those economic questions of land, housing, transit, with the need of the people for healthy conditions, and with their aspirations for beautiful surroundings and opportunities for a fuller and more social life" (Marquis, 1910).

In his *Town Planning Review* article of 1910, F.J. Marquis showed himself to be a philosophical radical. The feelings he expressed at that time were similar to those of the Coalition Government of the Second World War, and were encapsulated in the Beveridge Report. Speaking shortly after the Report was published, Sir William Beveridge stated that freedom from want was the aim of his report, but that want is only one of five specific evils to be attacked. Want, Disease, Ignorance, Squalor and Idleness, all must be destroyed.

The kind of society envisaged by the Beveridge Committee became a main objective of the Coalition Government and the subsequent Attlee and Churchill reconstruction governments.

Aneurin Bevan, Minister for Health in the Attlee Government, was perhaps the outstanding philosophical radical of the reconstruction period. He introduced a comprehensive National Health Service, with Henry Cohen, the Professor of Medicine at Liverpool University, as his principal adviser. And he saw that the maximum amount of local authority housing was built within the economic constraints of the immediate post-war years. The houses were designed to the high standards proposed in the Housing Manual, by the Parker Committee, which was guided by Judith Ledeboer, the architect chairman of the Housing Centre. She played the role which Raymond Unwin had filled for the Tudor Walters Committee during the First World War.

Bevan, the son of a Welsh miner, worked as a miner, attended the Central Labour College, and was first elected to Parliament at the age of 32. In the House of Commons he was held in respect as the only orator who could match Churchill in filling the House to overflowing. Churchill and Bevan were prominent opponents of the inept Baldwin and Chamberlain governments of the pre-war years. Churchill once described Chamberlain as a man who saw the world through the wrong end of a municipal sewer. Bevan's views are recorded in Hansard.

Backlash

The social, economic and physical reconstruction proposed and undertaken by the Churchill and Attlee governments was not without critics, both in the right wing press and in academic circles. "Throwing a planner in the works" was a typical *Evening Standard* headline. The voice of Friedrich August von Hayek, Professor of Economic Science and Statistics in the University of London, 1931-1950, was far more important. His influential *Road to Serfdom* was published in 1944, and his *Individualism and Economic Order* in 1948. He moved to the University of Chicago in 1950 as Professor of Social and Moral Science, where he joined Milton Friedman, who had been appointed Professor of Economics two years earlier. Friedman had started his professional life with the National Resources Committee, 1935-1937, a Roosevelt-appointed planning advisory body. After spending the following seven years in other government agencies he commenced his academic career in Columbia University. He won the Nobel Prize for Economic Science in 1976, and became the most influential economist of his time, espousing the free market, the privatisation of government enterprises, public assets and natural monopolies, and like von Hayek equating freedom with economic rationalism.

In comparison with the socio-economic world envisaged by the philosophical radicals of the 1830s and the 1950s, the economic rationalism of the 1980s and 1990s encouraged greed and selfishness, favoured the well-to-do, and created an unemployed underclass. Homeless people of all ages now live on the streets of the wealthier nations; a state of affairs that would never have been accepted by the compassionate society of the very much more difficult war and postwar years.

Affordable housing was being built by local authorities in reasonable quantities until the advent of Margaret Thatcher as Prime Minister (1979-1990). Her government set out to privatise public assets, mostly services and natural monopolies, including local authority housing. It was as if she was determined to savage the socio-economic reforms effected by the Churchill and Attlee led philosophical radicals of the Second World War. Some 23,000 affordable local authority dwellings were built in the year 1993, compared with the 200,000 and 300,000 per year achieved by the Attlee government and the second Churchill government. Unfettered market forces are now the order of the day, and they carry the seeds of both dynamism and disaster.

In reviewing *The Empty Raincoat,* a book by Charles Handy, Peter Kellner had this to say (Kellner, 1994). "Capitalism – and especially British capitalism – still has its biggest enemy to confront: its own failings. What is happening in our mature societies," he writes, "is much more fundamental, confusing and distressing than I had expected. Too many people are losers: jobless, alien and without decent homes. Capitalism has proved more rigid and divisive, and governments more stupid than Handy had hoped earlier in his long career as chronicler, analyst, management theorist (and Chairman of the Royalty Society of Arts Council)."

In Handy's view, capitalism in general, and the profit motive in particular, should be means to an end, not ends in themselves. As early as 1776, in *An Inquiry into the Nature and Causes of the Wealth of Nations,* Adam Smith was the first to formulate principles of political economy, saying that a stable and prosperous society was based on 'sympathy' – meaning a moral duty to have regard for your fellow human beings. That was the philosophy motivating the Churchill and Attlee Governments, and it led to compassionate planning. The time is ripe for a new generation of philosophical radicals to enter and hold sway in the House of Commons.

References

Bauer, Catherine, 1934, *Modern Housing*, George Allen and Unwin, London.

Simey, Margaret, 1992, *Charity Rediscovered*, Liverpool University Press.

Frazer, W.M., 1947, *Duncan of Liverpool*, Hamish Hamilton Medical Books, London.

Lancaster, Osbert, 1939, *From Pillar to Post*, John Murray, London.

Howard, Ebenezer, 1902, *Garden Cities of Tomorrow*, Swan Sonnenschein and Co., London.

Hyde, Francis, 1947, *Utilitarian Town Planning*, Town Planning Review, Vol. XIX, No. 3, Liverpool University Press.

Stephenson, Gordon, *Architecture, Town Planning and Civic Design*, 1985, Town Planning Review, Vol. 56, No. 2, Liverpool University Press.

Wakefield, E.G., 1849, *The Art of Colonisation*, J.W. Parker, London.

Hight, James and Straubel, C.R., 1957, *A History of Canterbury*, Vol. 1, Whitcombe and Tombs, Christchurch.

Hutchings, Alan, and Bunker, Raymond, 1986, *With Conscious Purpose*, A History of Town Planning in South Australia, Wakefield Press, Adelaide.

Bacon, Edmund, N., 1967, *Design of Cities*, The Viking Press, New York.

Reddaway, T.F., 1939, *The Rebuilding of London After the Great Fire*, Town Planning Review, Vol. XVIII, No. 3, University of Liverpool.

Geddes Patrick, 1915, *Cities in Evolution:* an Introduction to the Town Planning Movement and to the Study of Civics, Williams and Norgate, London.

De Soissons, Louis and Kenyon, Arthur, 1927, *Site Planning in Practice at Welwyn Garden City*, Ernest Benn, London.

Final Report of the New Towns Committee, July, 1946, Cmnd. 6876, HMSO, London. The Interim and Second Interim Reports were published in March and April, 1946.

Report of the Committee on Qualifications of Planners, Chairman Sir George Schuster, 1950, Cmnd 8059, HMSO, London.

Unwin, Raymond, 1909, *Town Planning in Practice,* T. Fisher, Unwin, London.

Stein, Clarence, 1951, *Toward New Towns for America*, Liverpool University Press.

Mumford, Lewis, 1938, *The Culture of Cities*, Harcourt Brace, New York.

State of New York, *Report of the Commission of Housing and Regional Planning to Governor Alfred E. Smith*, Chairman, Clarence S. Stein, Adviser, Henry Wright, 1926, J.B. Lyon & Co., Albany, New York.

The Regional Survey of New York and its Environs, Chairman Thomas Adams, 1929, Russell Sage Foundation, New York.

Royal Commission on the Distribution of the Industrial Population, Chairman Sir Montague Barlow, 1940, Cmnd 6153, HMSO, London.

Forshaw, J.H. and Abercrombie, Patrick, 1943, *County of London Plan*, MacMillan and Co., London.

Abercrombie, Patrick, 1944, *Greater London Plan*, HMSO, London.

Committee on Land Utilisation in Rural Areas, Lord Justice Scott, Chairman, 1942, Cmnd 6378, HMSO, London.

Expert Committee on Compensation and Betterment, Final Report, Mr Justice Uthwatt, Chairman, 1942, Cmnd 6386, HMSO, London.

Second Report of the Greater London Regional Planning Committee, Technical Adviser, Sir Raymond Unwin, 1933, Knapp, Drewett and Sons, London.

Karsh, Yousuf, 1959, *Portraits of Greatness*, University of Toronto Press.

Marquis, F.J. 1910, *Some Sociological Aspects of Town Planning*, Town Planning Review, Vol. 1, No. 1, Liverpool University Press.

Kellner, Peter, July, 1994, book review, *RSA Journal*, Royal Society of Arts, London.